To Jake and Juliette, my little yogis!
Special thanks to my photographer Jacqueline Eucare
My editor Amie McCracken,
My talented illustrator Erica Volpe,
And all of the incredible parents and children who helped make this work so special.

Illustrations by Erica Volpe
Interior Design by Amie McCracken

ISBN: 978-0-692-94468-4

Yogaventure

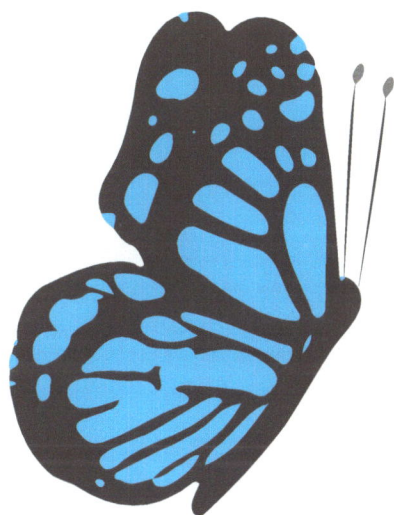

Written by Jillian Amodio
Illustrated by Erica Volpe

What is Yoga?

The word Yoga can be interpreted to mean unity. It refers to unity of mind, body, and spirit. People who practice yoga are called yogis. Yoga originated over 5,000 years ago. That's a really long time! It first originated in India. While most people are familiar with the physical poses (asana), there are actually 8 limbs of yoga. Yoga is not a religion. It is more of a lifestyle or a guide to healthy living.

Who can do yoga?

Yoga is for everyone. Anyone anywhere can practice yoga. You don't have to be incredibly flexible or super fit. People of any age and any skill level can find yoga to be enjoyable and beneficial. Yoga can be modified to fit the individual needs of every person. A recent study showed that over 20 million people practice yoga in the United States alone! It is not surprising that so many people turn to yoga. The benefits are unending.

What can yoga do for you?

Practicing yoga is beneficial for physical, emotional, and mental health. It inspires, uplifts, and promotes well-rounded living. It can reduce stress and improve overall health. Yoga is great for focus and can increase flexibility and build strength. Practicing yoga can help with your overall mood and can even prevent and manage many diseases and health conditions. Yoga promotes positive living and compassion towards yourself and others. Yoga does all this and more! Plus, it's really fun!

Are you ready to meet some new friends?
Come on! Let's go on a Yogaventure!

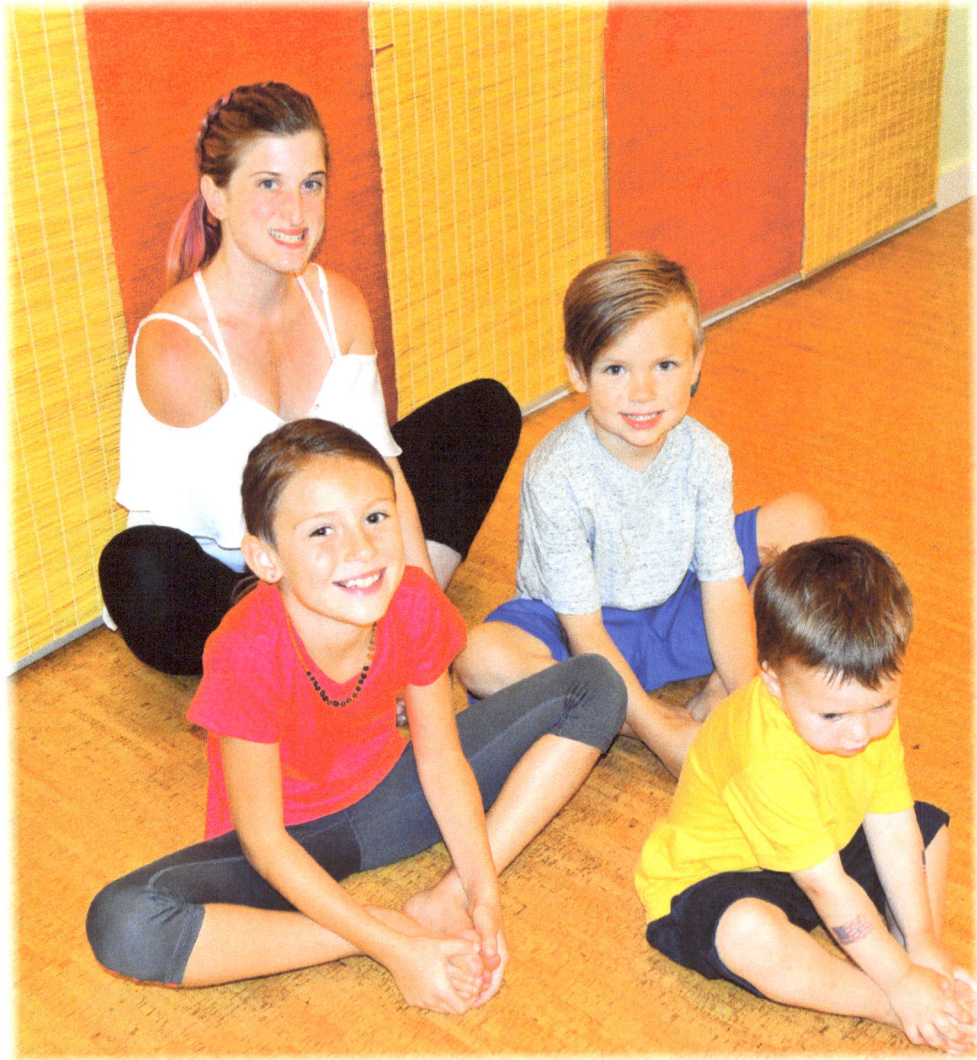

Sitting up nice and tall, imagine you are a beautiful butterfly. Bring the bottoms of your feet together to form brightly colored wings. Continue with your deep breaths as you gently flap your wings up and down. Close your eyes and imagine yourself flying from flower to flower.

Butterfly pose is good for improving posture and stretching the inner thighs.

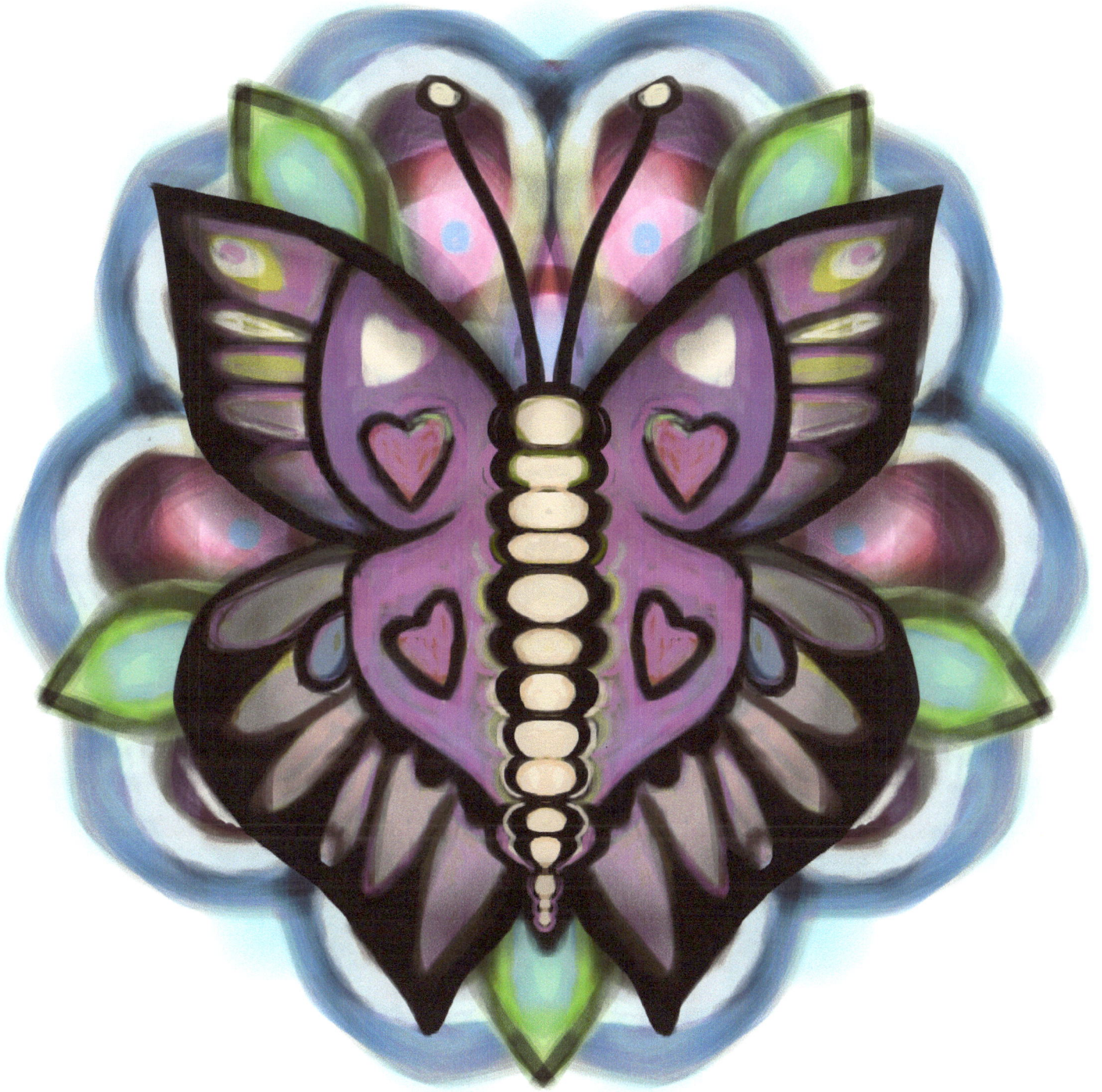

One day we decided to go for a walk.
We met a butterfly, and just stopped to talk,
and that butterfly, oh that butterfly,
that butterfly looked like this.

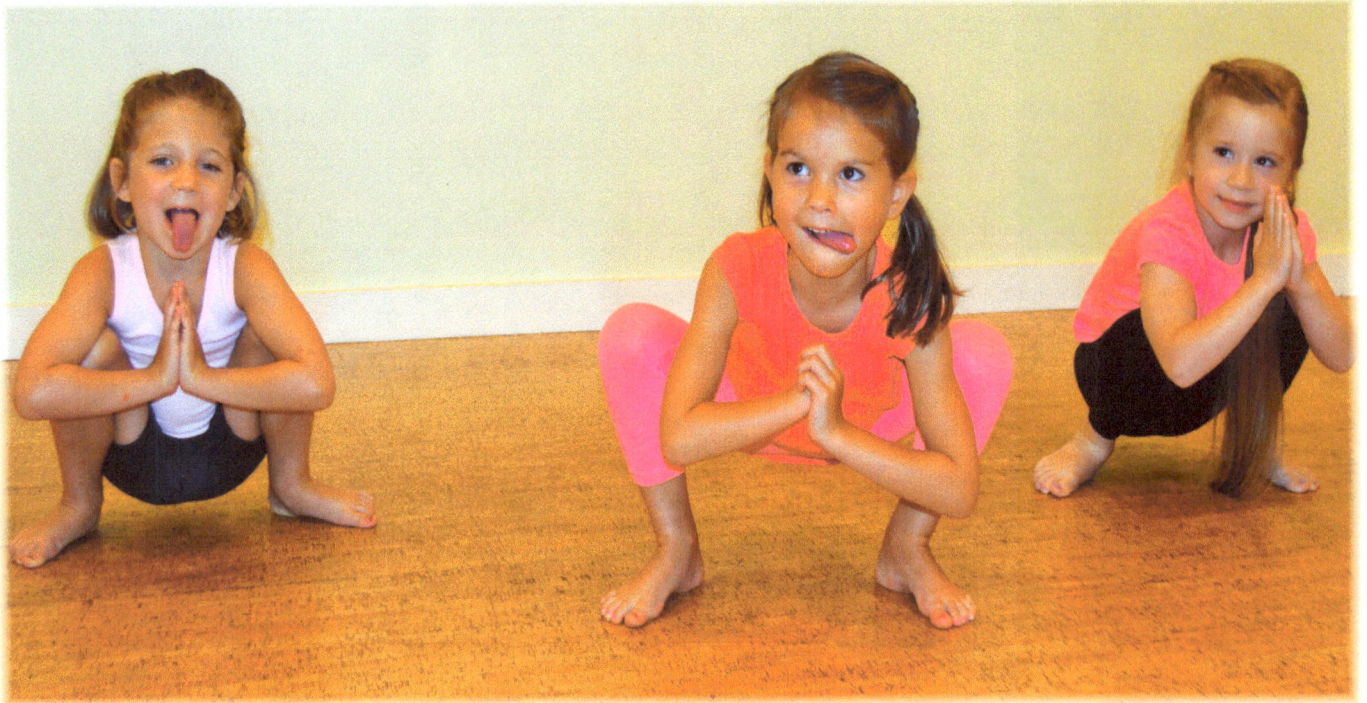

Spread your frog legs wide and bend your knees to squat on your lily pad. Put your froggy arms in between your knees and imagine yourself calmly sitting on your lily pad just waiting for a yummy fly to cross your path. Now take a big froggy jump and say Rrribit!

This pose, traditionally known as Garland pose, is good for bringing a sense of calm and balance. It can also be helpful for digestion.

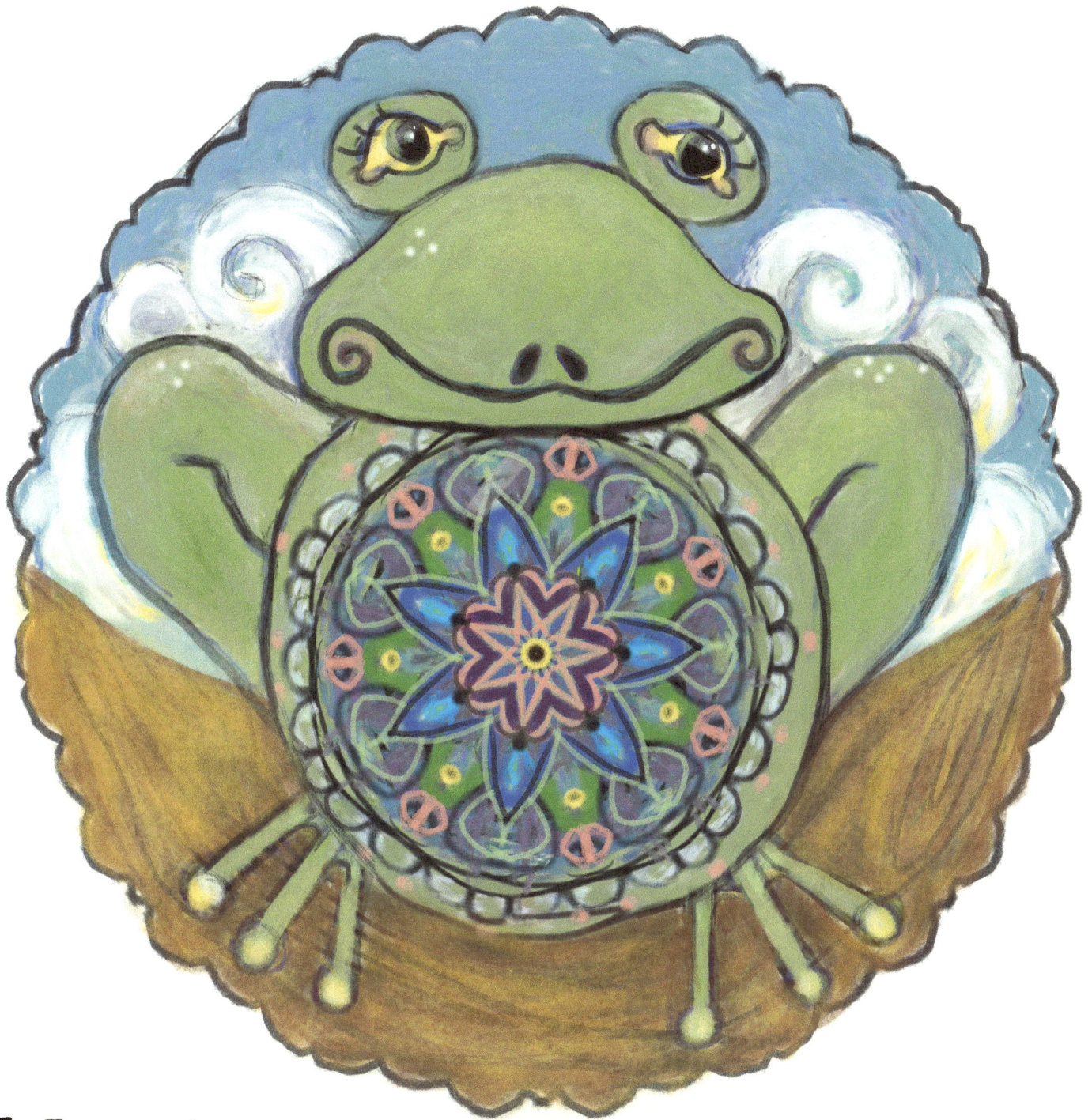

We continued our walk and we met a frog.
He was sitting on a wet and slippery log,
and that little frog, oh that little frog,
that frog he looked like this.

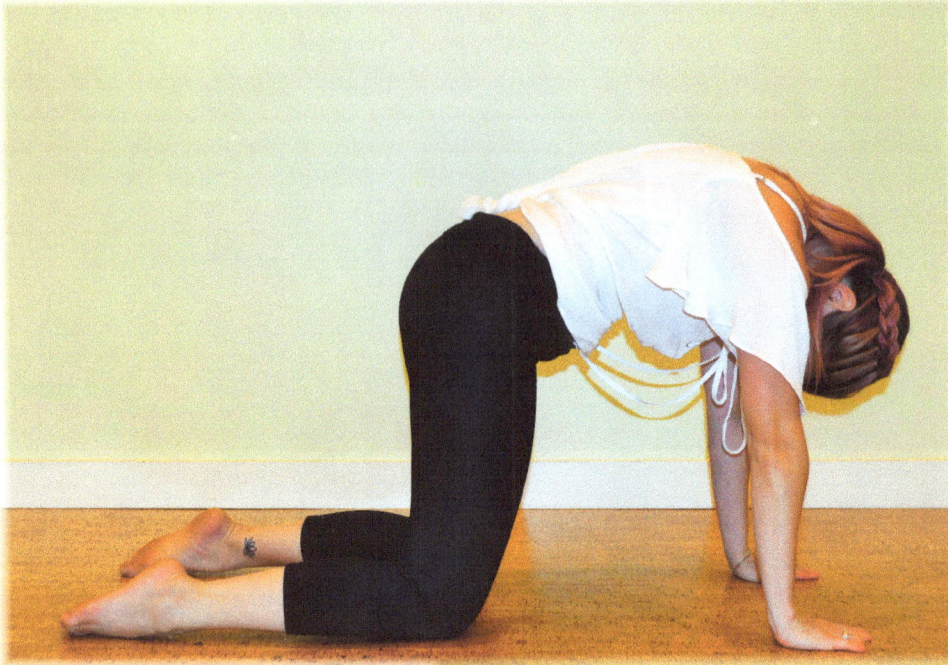

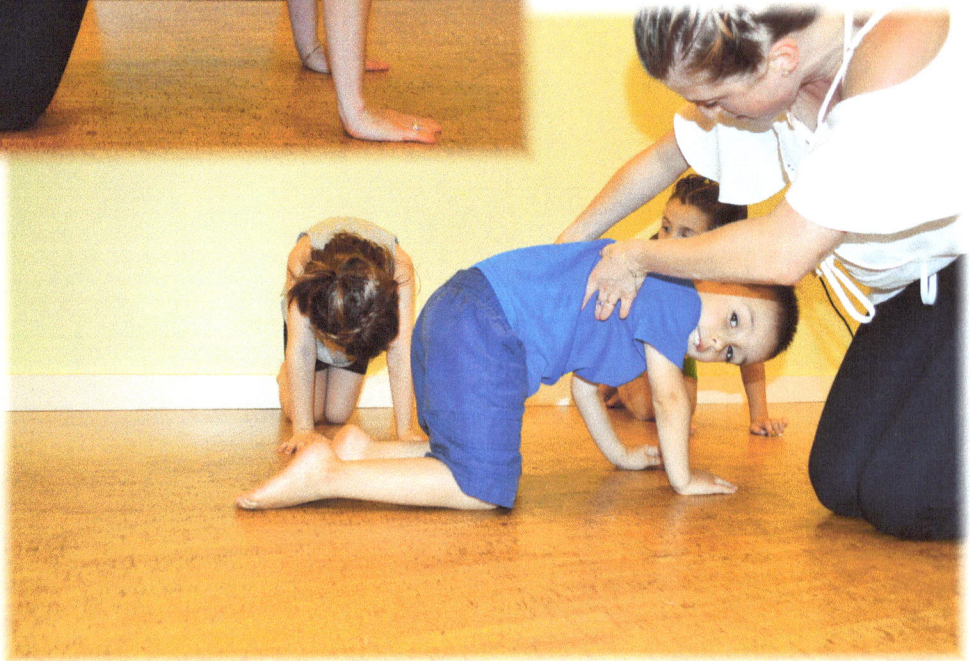

Pretend you are a cat on your hands and knees. As you breathe in look up to the sky with a big cat stretch. As you breath out, arch your back and say Meow!

Cat pose is good for stretching the muscles in the back and massaging the internal organs for proper function.

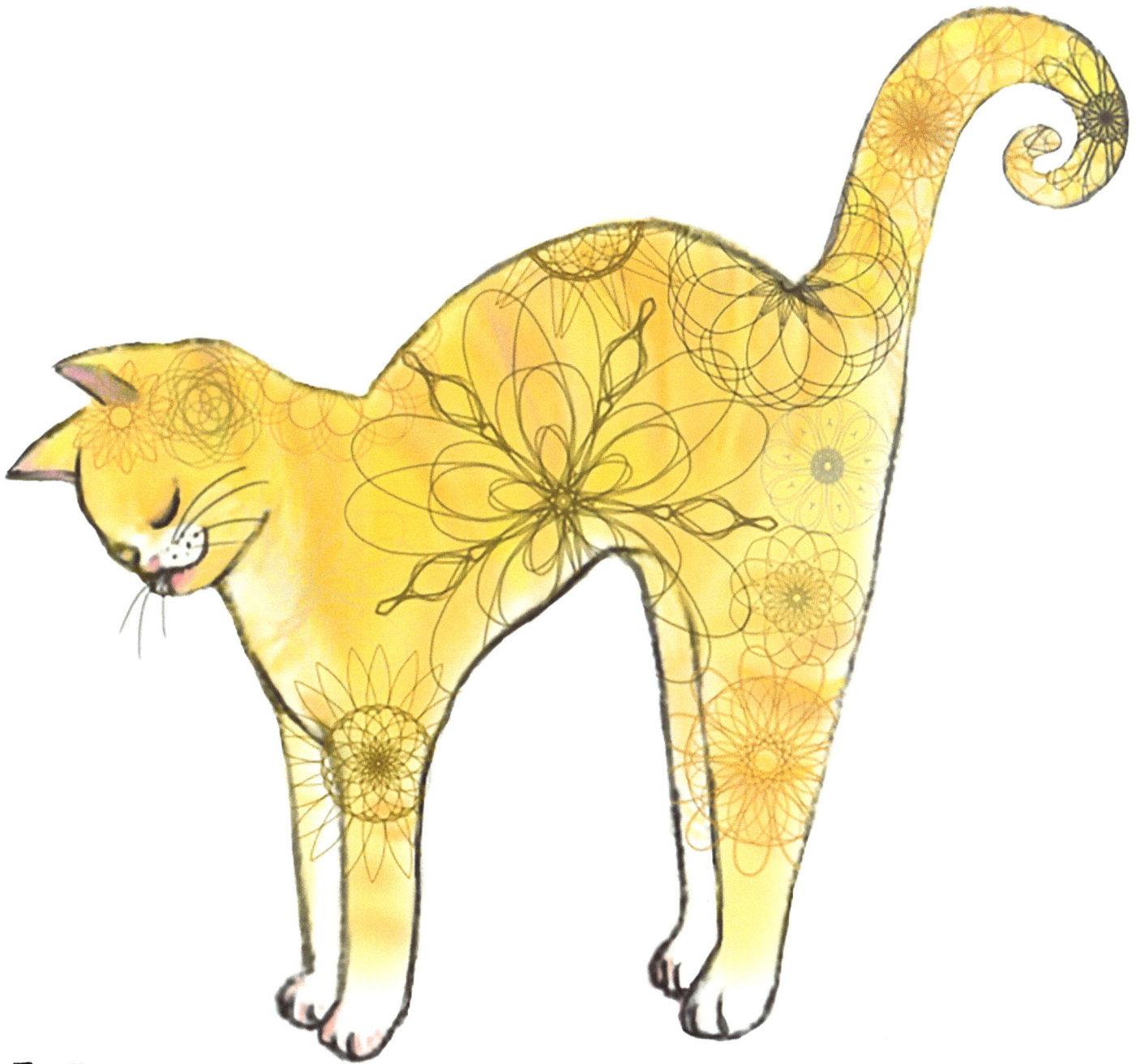

We said "Goodbye Mr. Frog, we have somewhere to be at." That's when we met a furry little kitty cat, and that little cat, oh that little cat, that cat she looked like this.

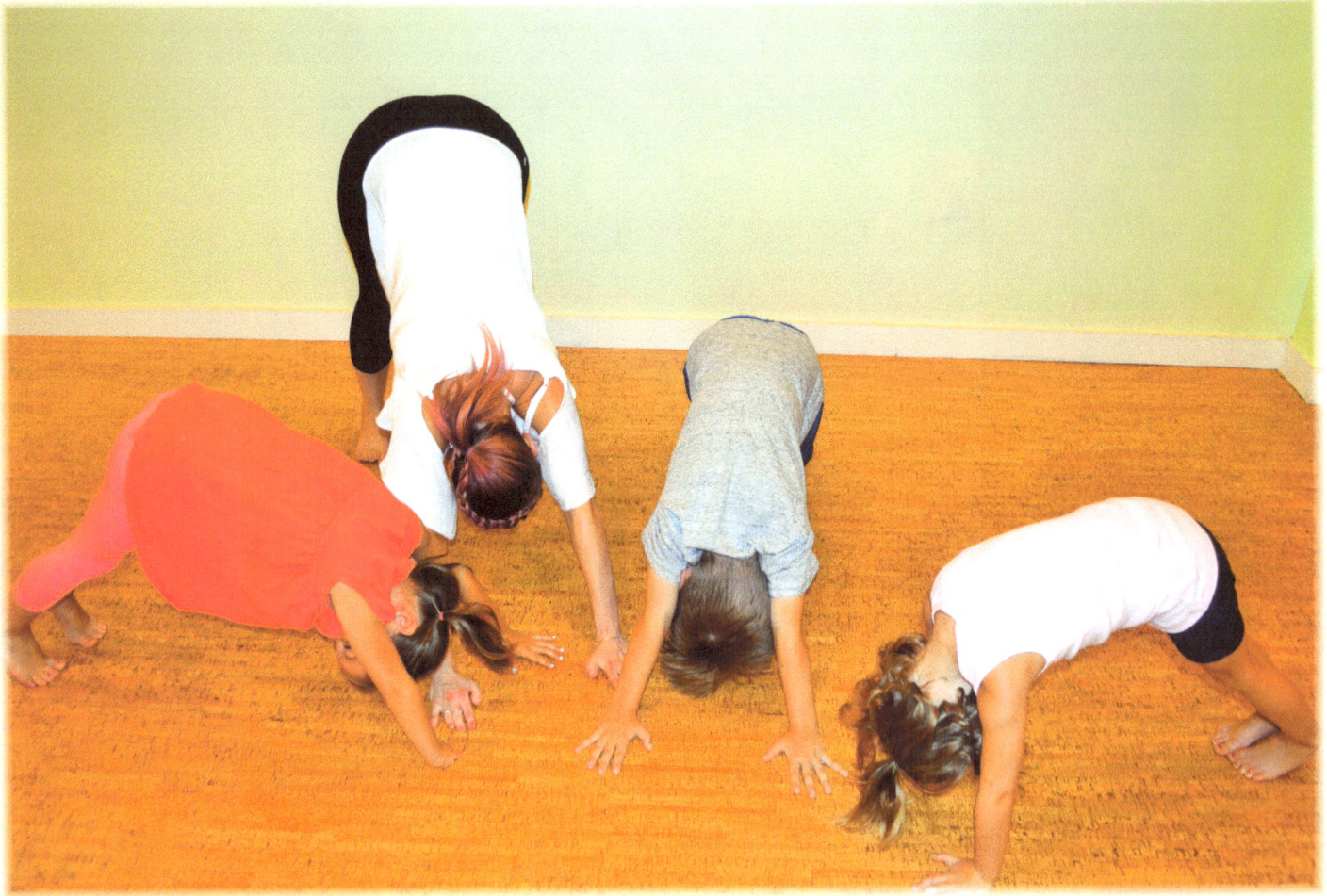

Lift your hips towards the sky like a puppy stretching after a nap. Wag your tail and say Woof woof! Release back down to hands and knees when ready.

Down Dog is beneficial for stretching the hamstrings, strengthening the arms, and can aid in relieving stress and fatigue.

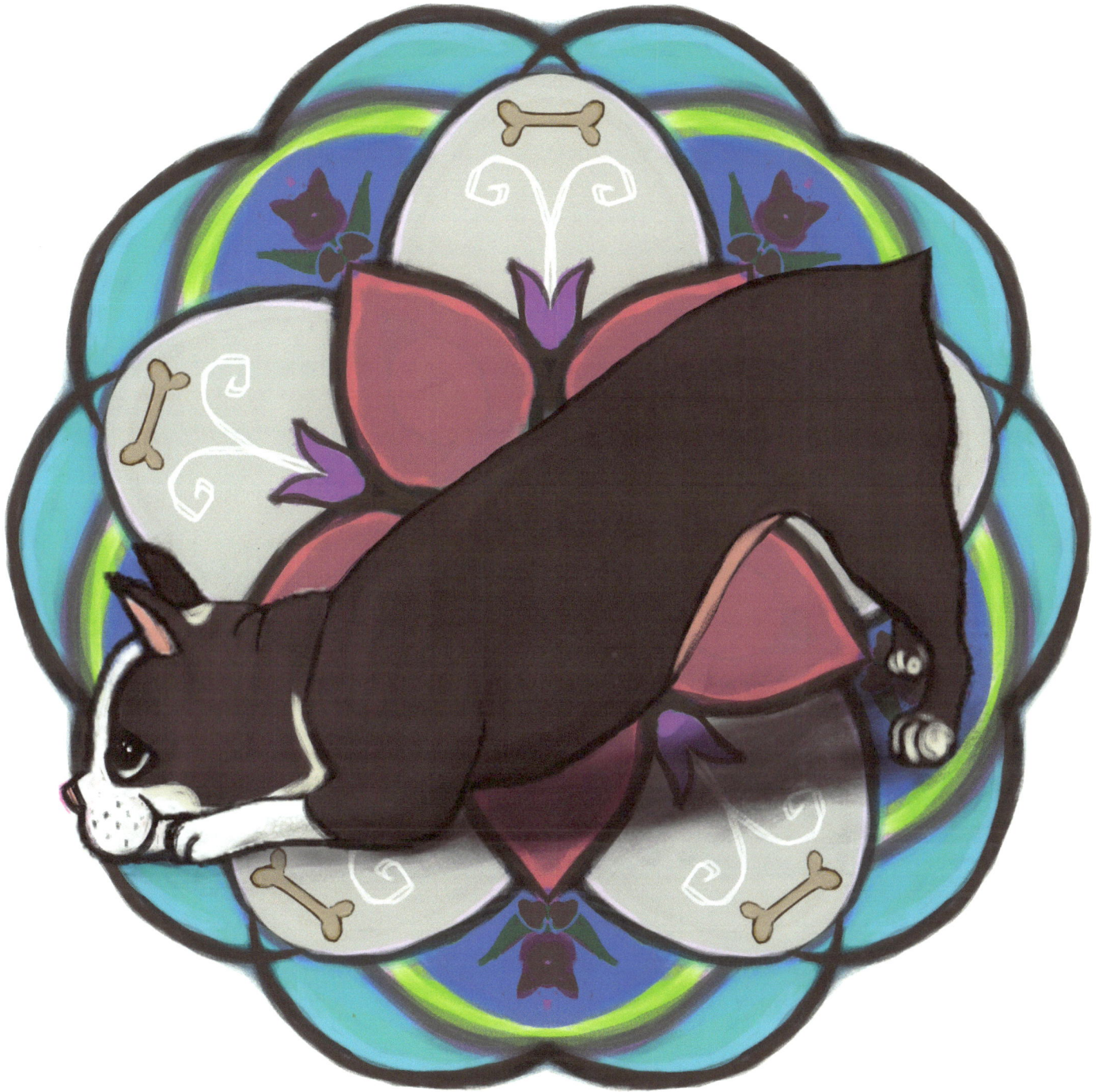

As we were chatting with the cat,
she took off in a jog. That's when we noticed
a little brown dog, and that little dog,
oh that little dog, that dog he looked like this.

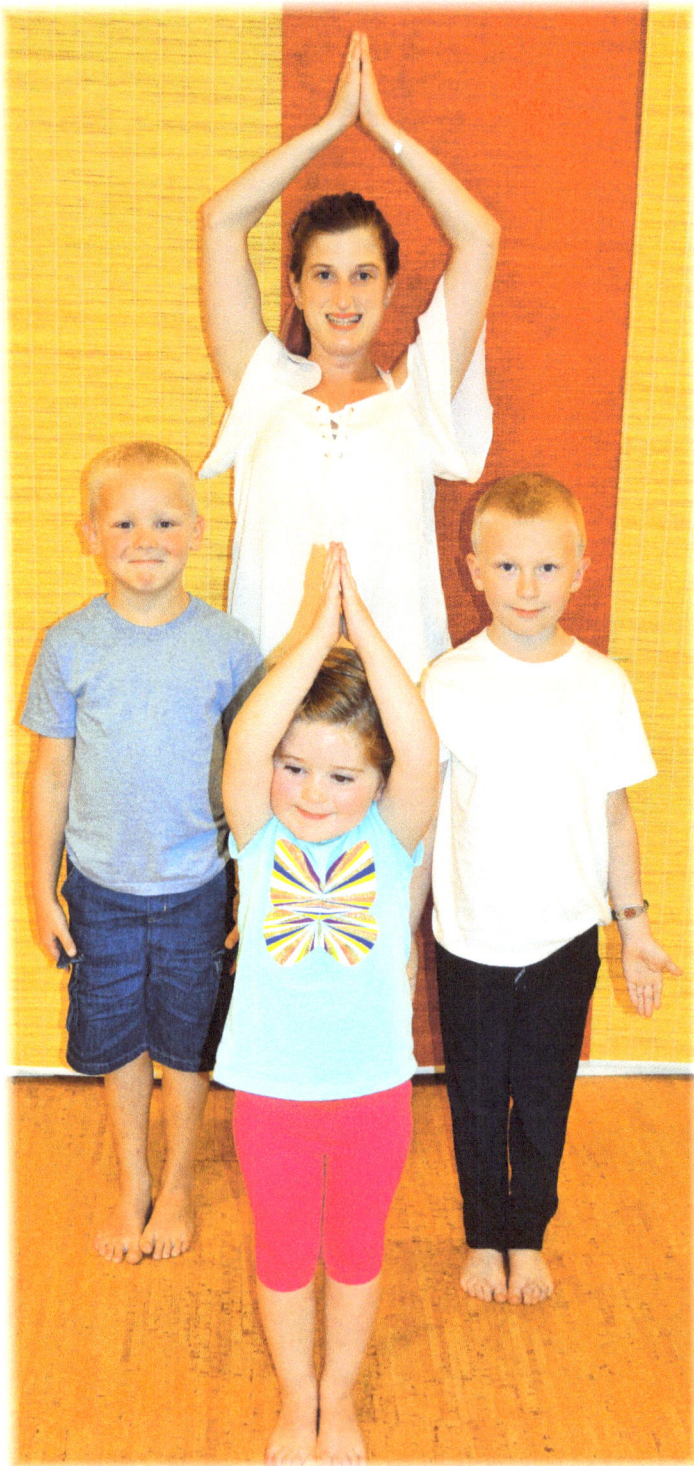

Stand up as tall as you can and pretend your feet are the strong base of a giant mountain. The top of your head is like the peak of a mountain reaching straight up into the clouds. Wow! Look at the view from up here!

Mountain pose is a great foundation pose. It encourages good posture and strengthens the core muscles.

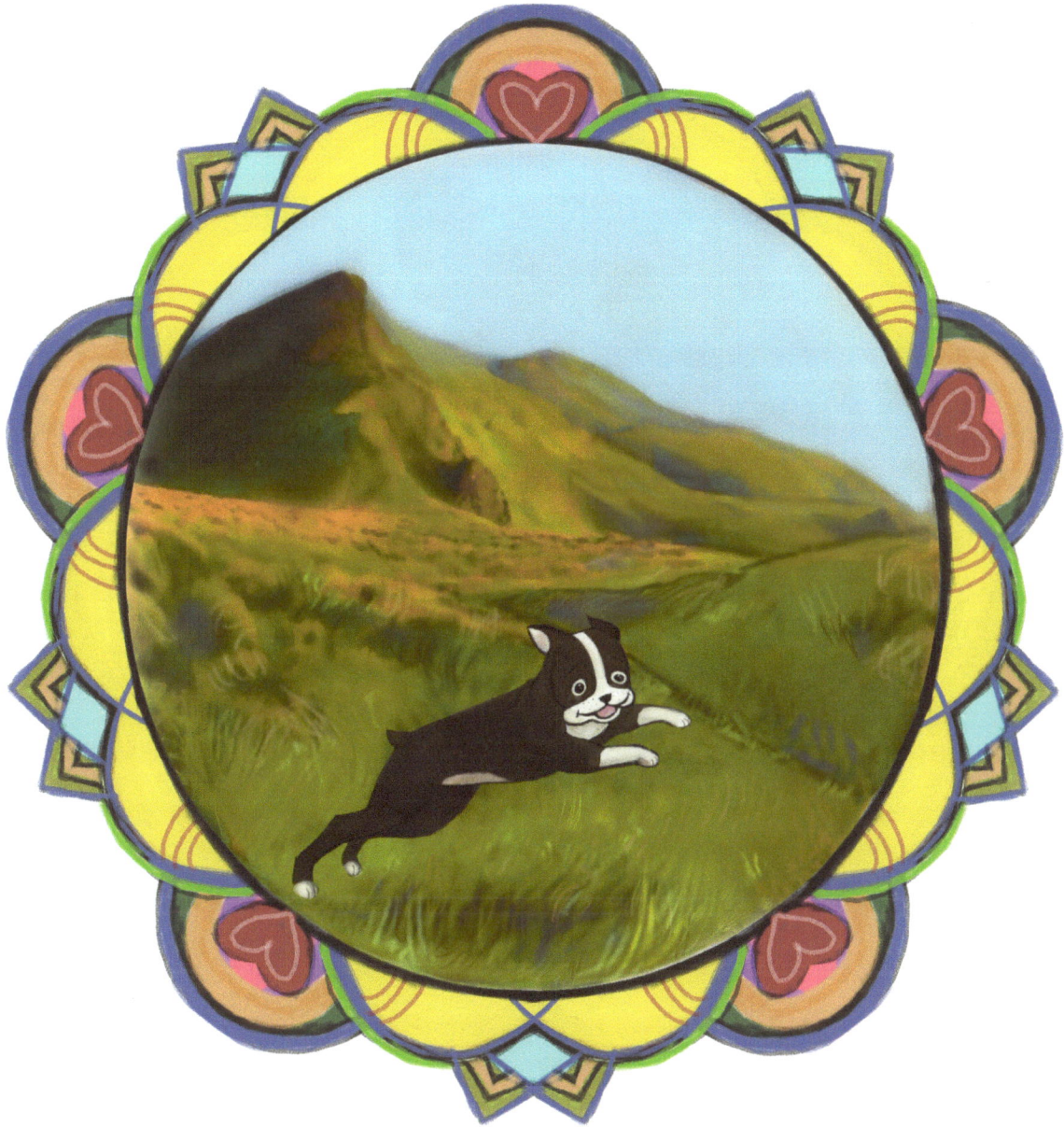

We got up with the dog and he ran nonstop.
He took us up to a big mountaintop,
and that mountaintop, oh that mountaintop,
that mountaintop looked like this.

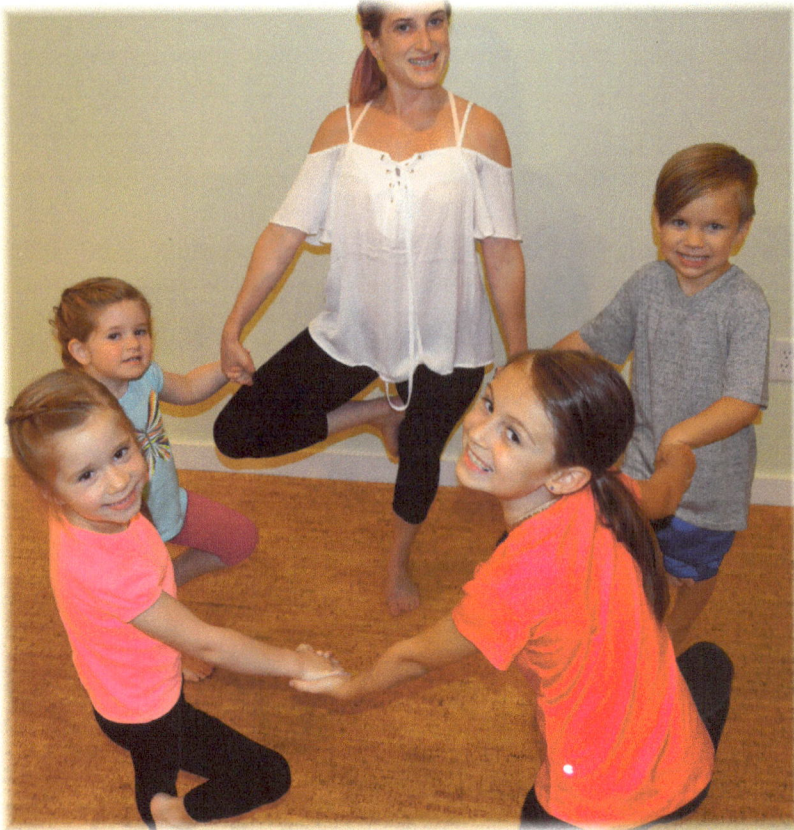

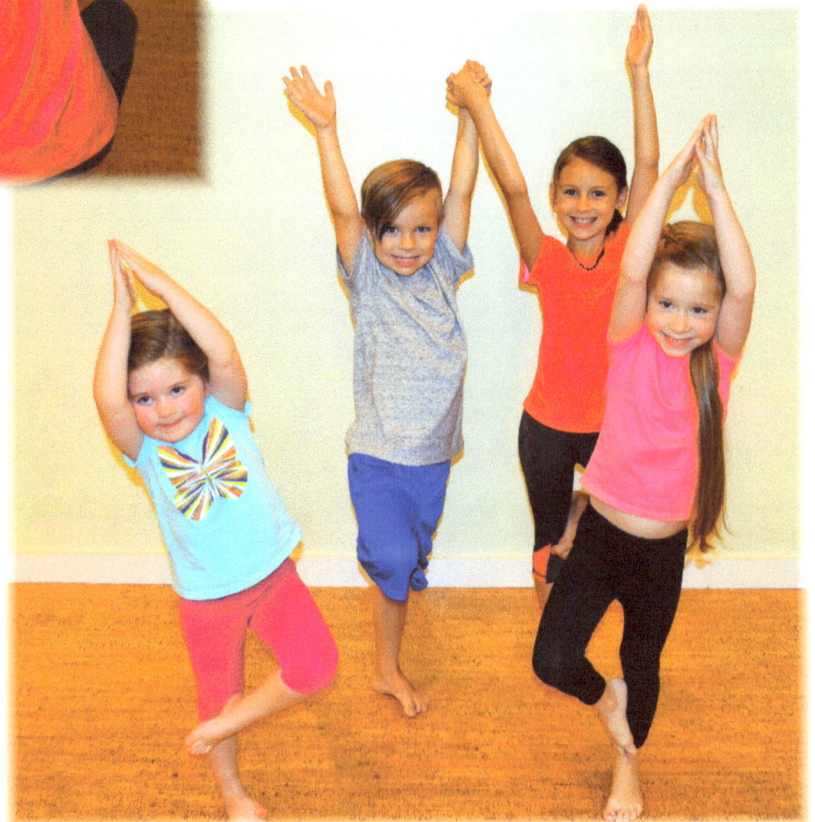

Begin to lift one foot and find balance on the other leg. If you feel balanced, lift your foot and rest it on your calf or even inner thigh. Let's pretend to be trees swaying in the wind. Move your arms and pretend that you are sprouting branches. Then set your foot down and try this with other side.

Tree pose encourages good balance and focus.

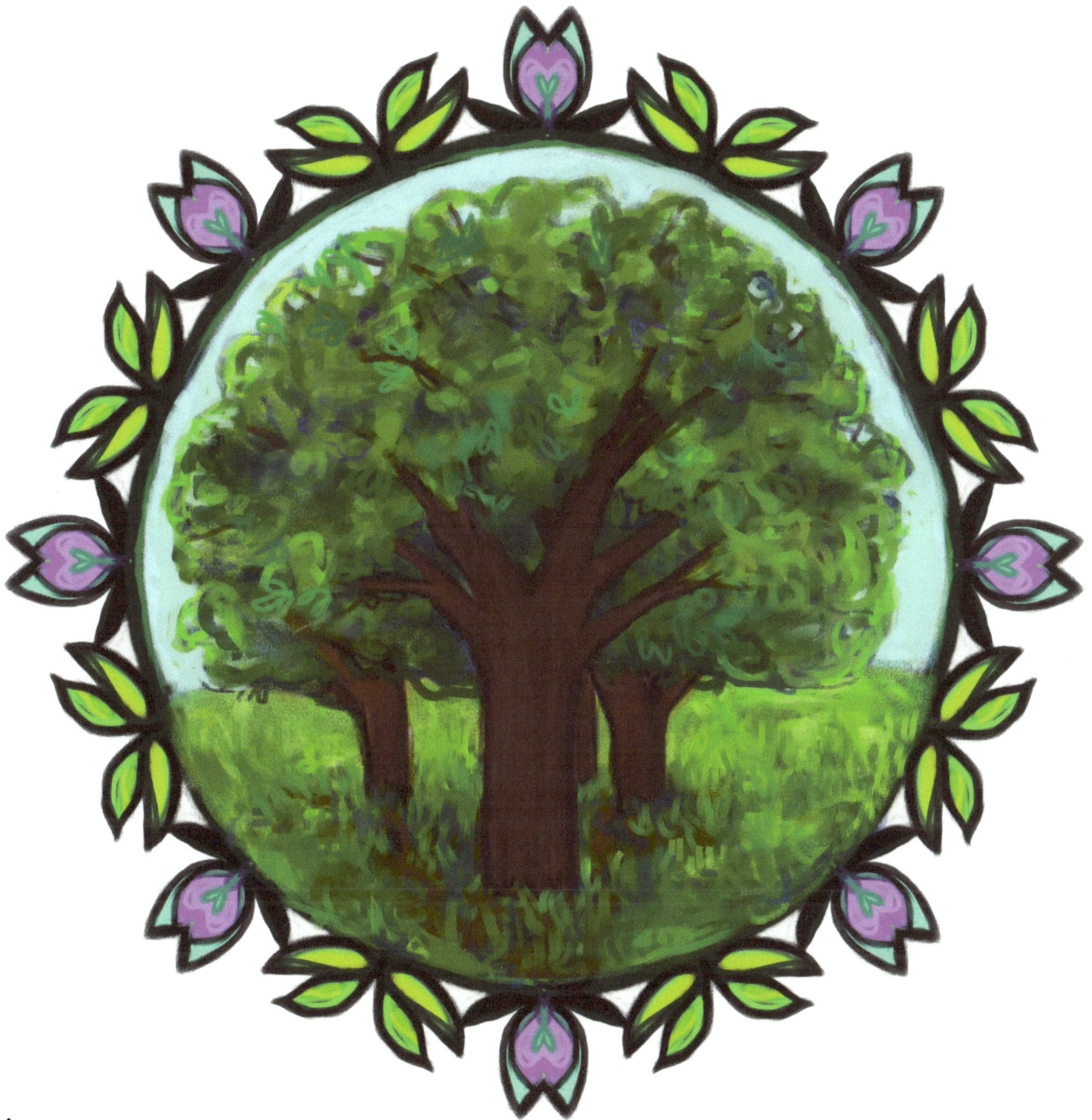

As we were coming down the mountain,
it was quite hard to see. For everywhere
we looked, we were surrounded by trees,
and those big tall trees, oh those big tall trees,
those trees they looked like this.

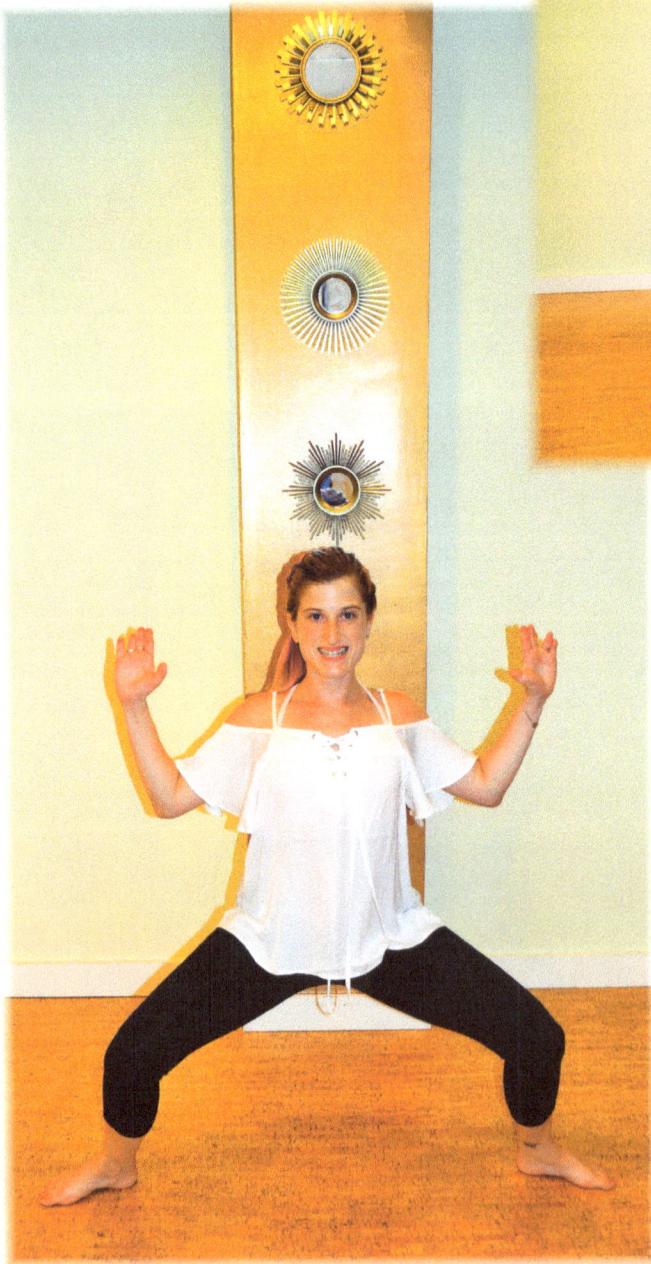

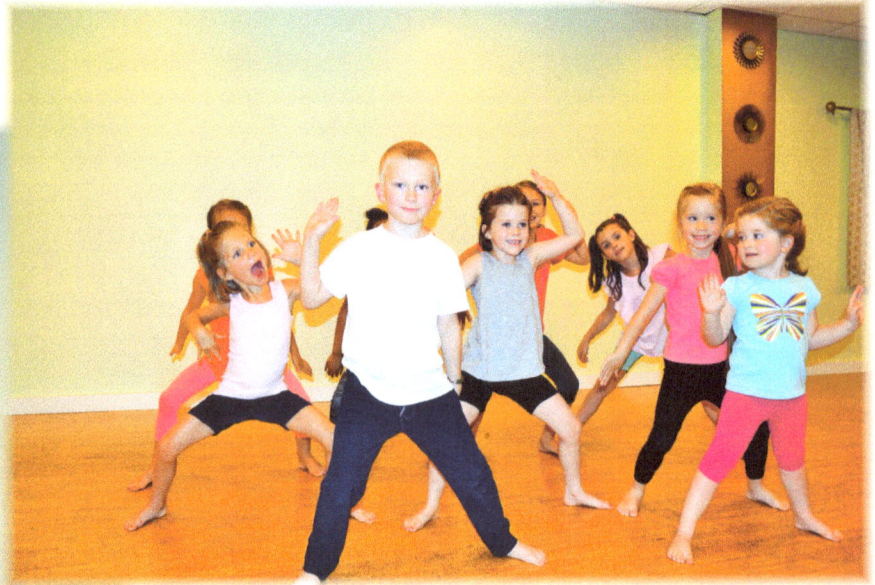

Now spread your feet wide apart. Raise your arms up like robot arms with your fingertips pointing to the sky. Princes and Princesses love to dance at their fancy parties. Can you show me your coolest robot move? Bend your knees and move your arms up and down.

This pose is known as Goddess pose and is good for stretching the hips and building core and leg strength.

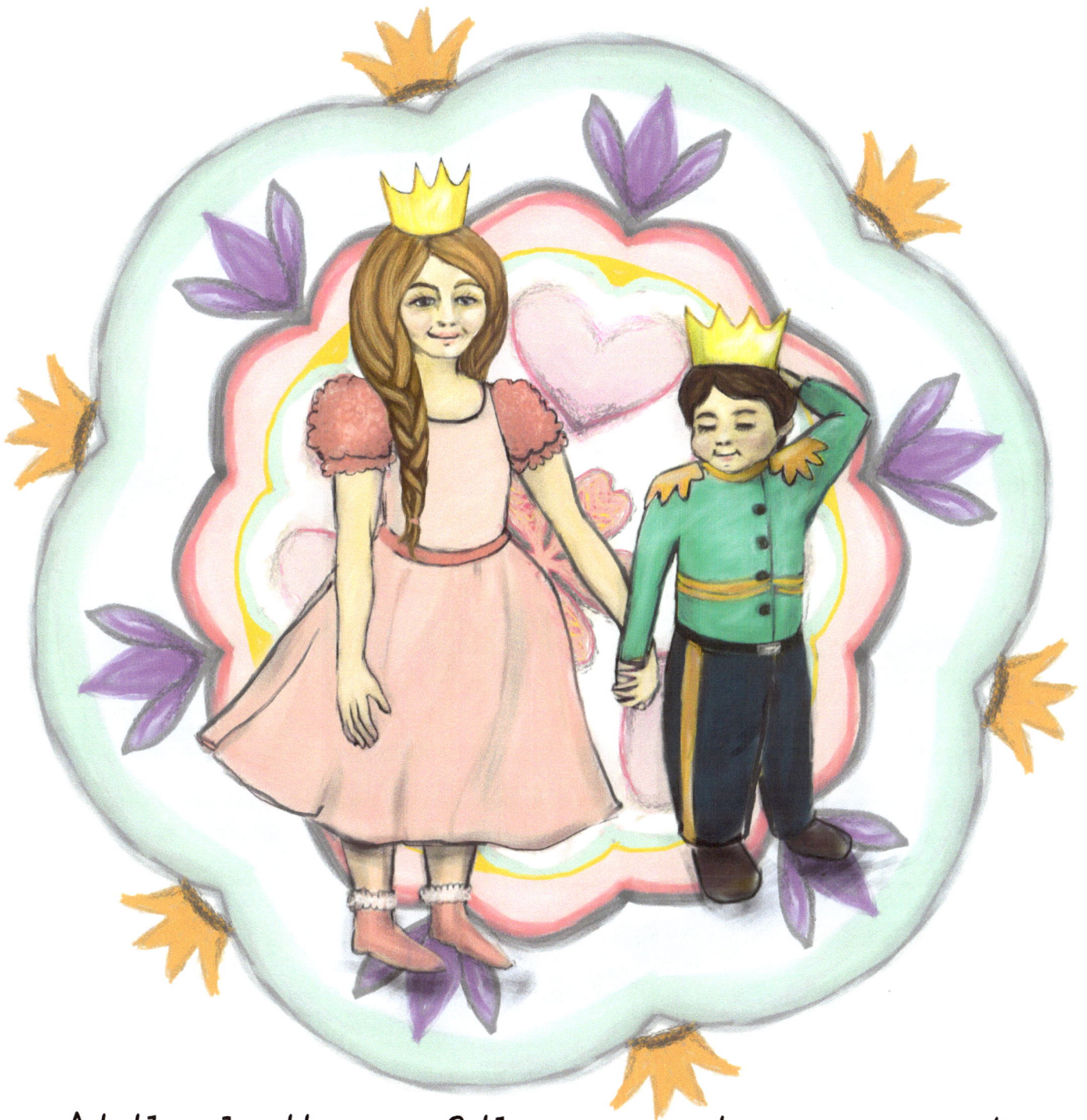

At the bottom of the mountain we met
a prince and a princess. He wore a crown,
and she a pretty pink dress,
and that little prince and his princess,
they both danced like this.

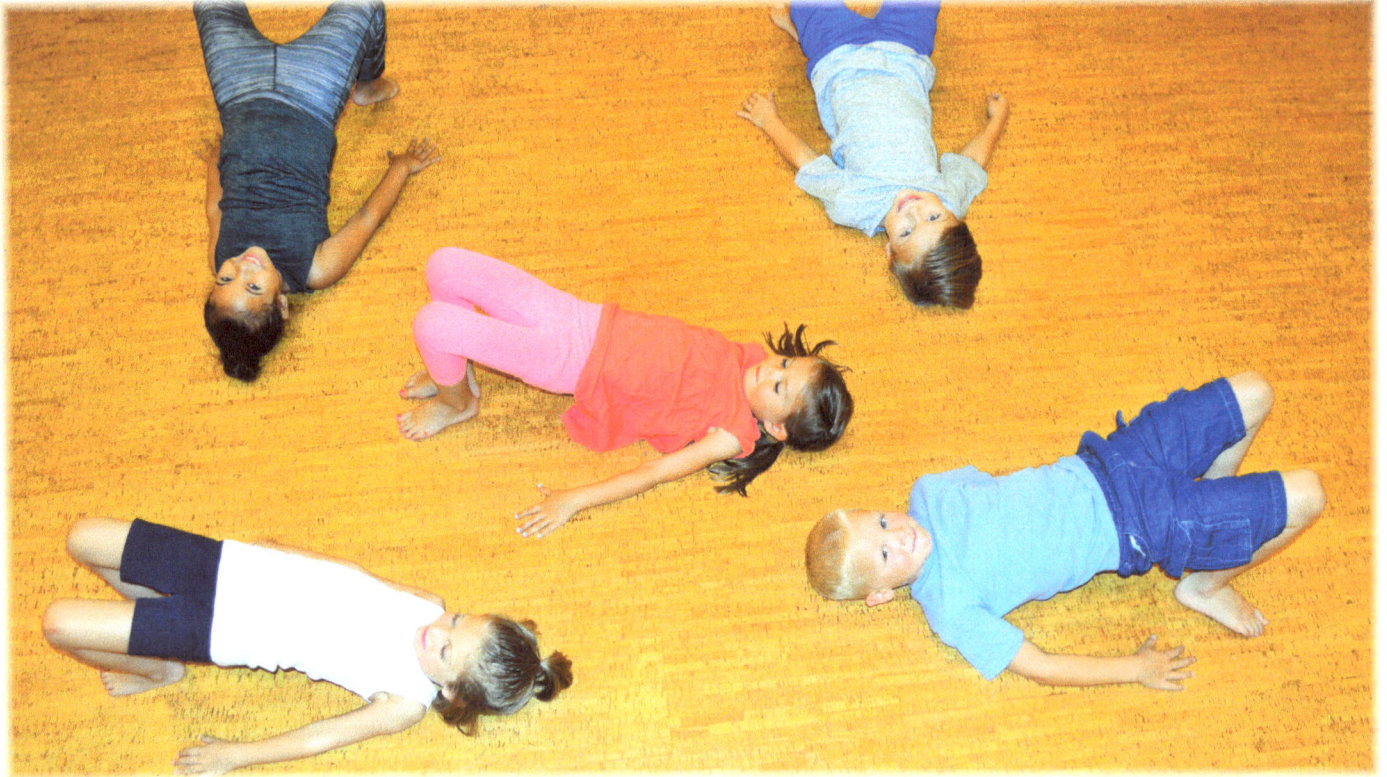

Lie on your back with your feet on the floor. Imagine you are a bridge and a boat is getting ready to pass under you. Here comes the boat! Breathe in and lift your drawbridge up up up! Great! The boat has passed, lower your bridge all the way back down.

Bridge pose aides in digestion, improves circulation, and strengthens the back and legs.

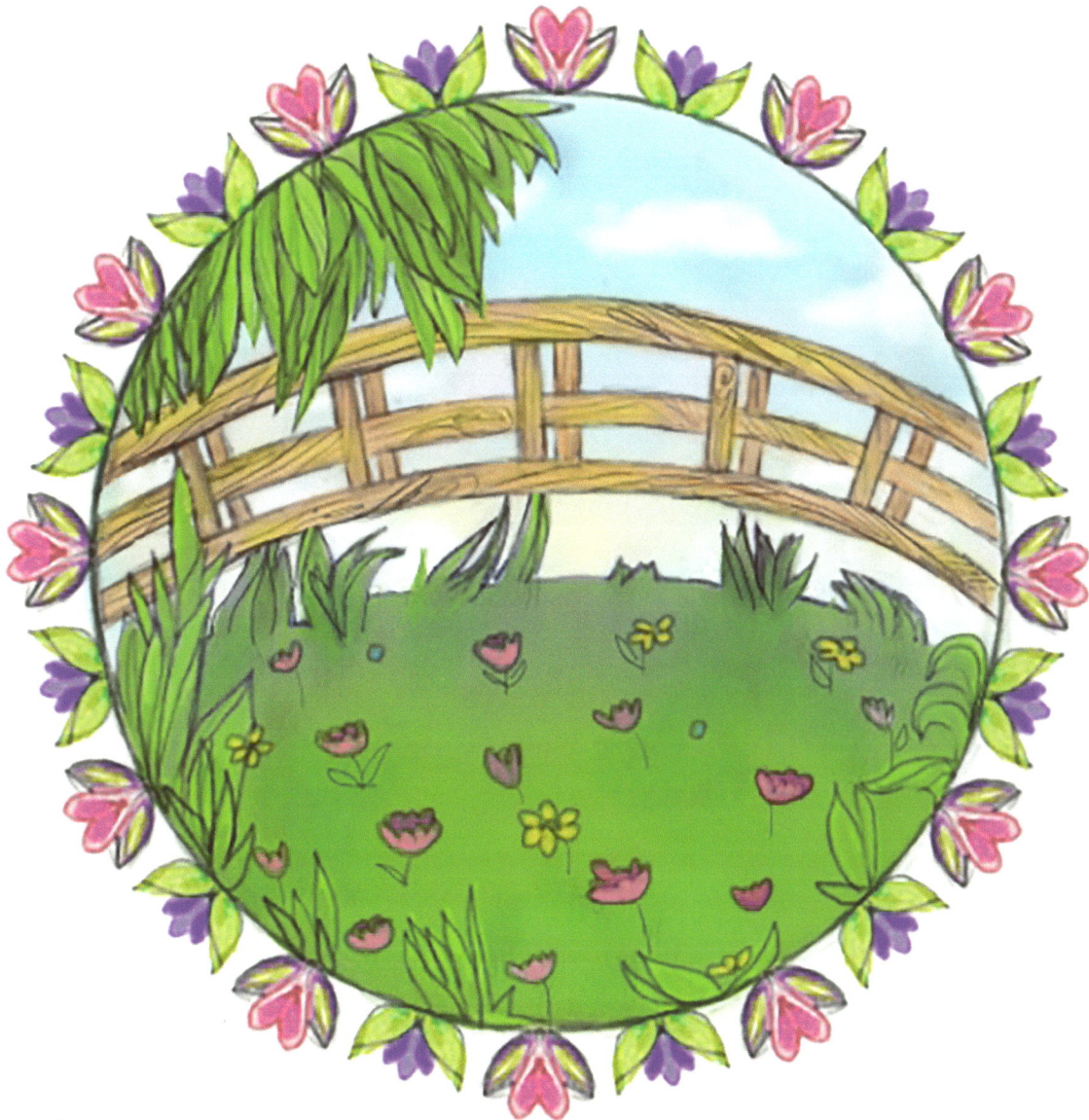

They took us to a bridge that led over a stream.
It was as pretty as a picture in a
beautiful dream, and that pretty bridge,
oh that pretty bridge,
that bridge it looked like this.

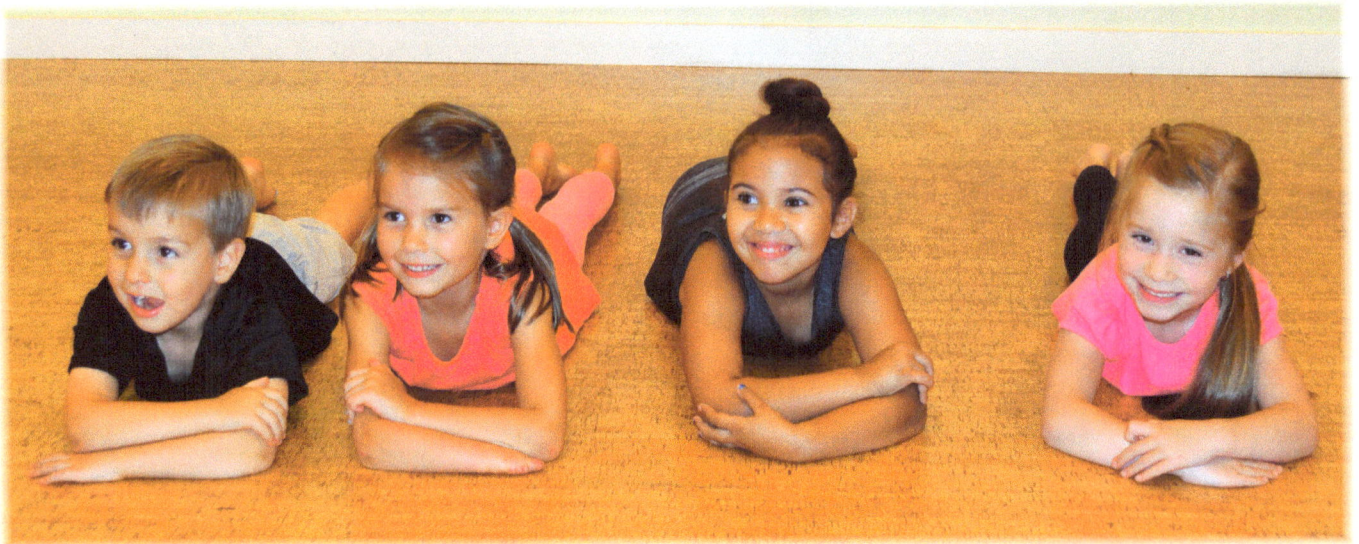

Roll over on your belly and stretch out like a lazy crocodile. Fold your arms in front of you. Are you a sleepy crocodile resting his head, or are you a sneaky crocodile peeking your head out of the water looking for lunch?

Crocodile pose is calming and encourages rest and relaxation.

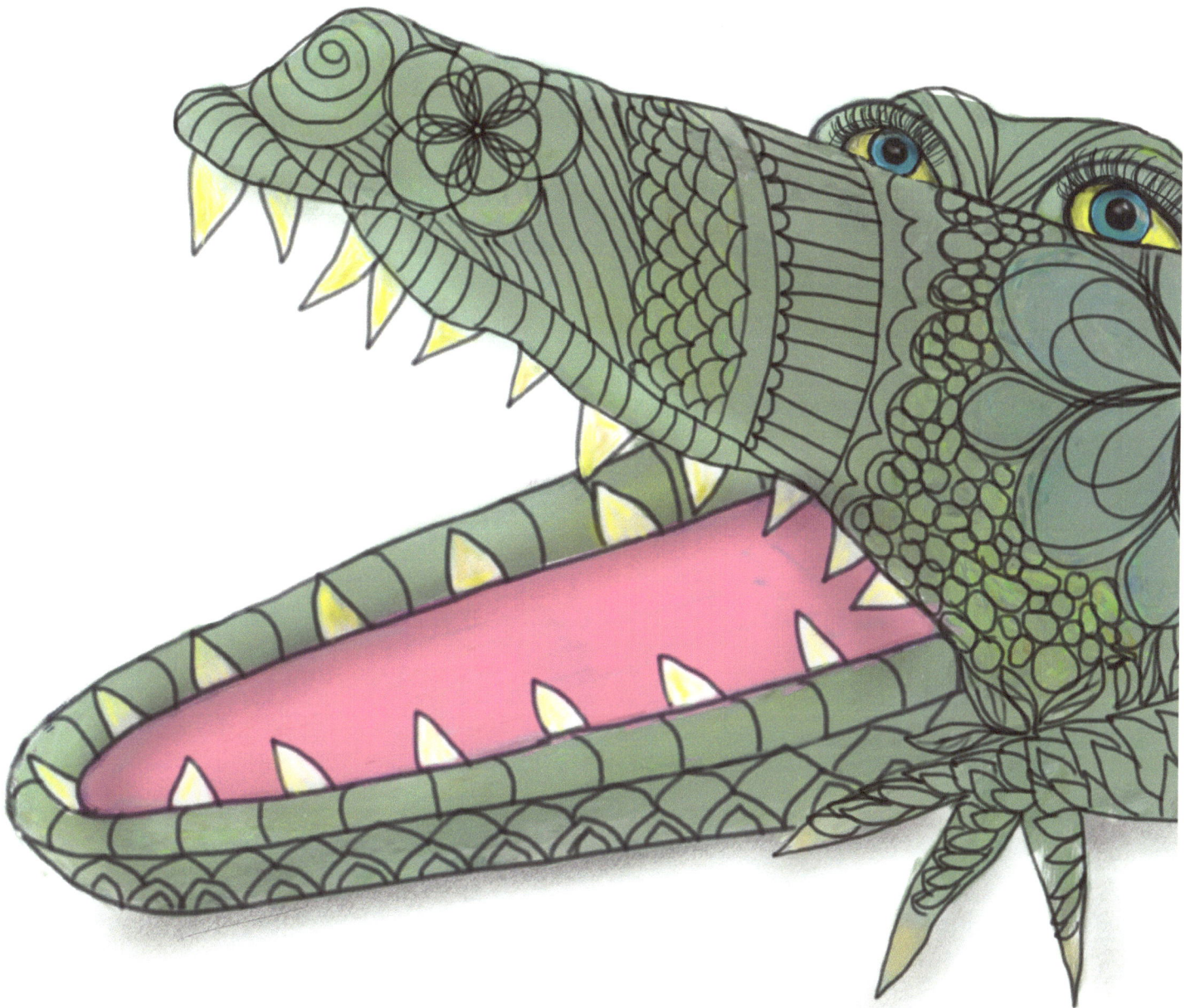

We crossed over the bridge
and stared for a while.
When what did we see, but a big crocodile,
and that crocodile, oh that crocodile,
that crocodile looked like this.

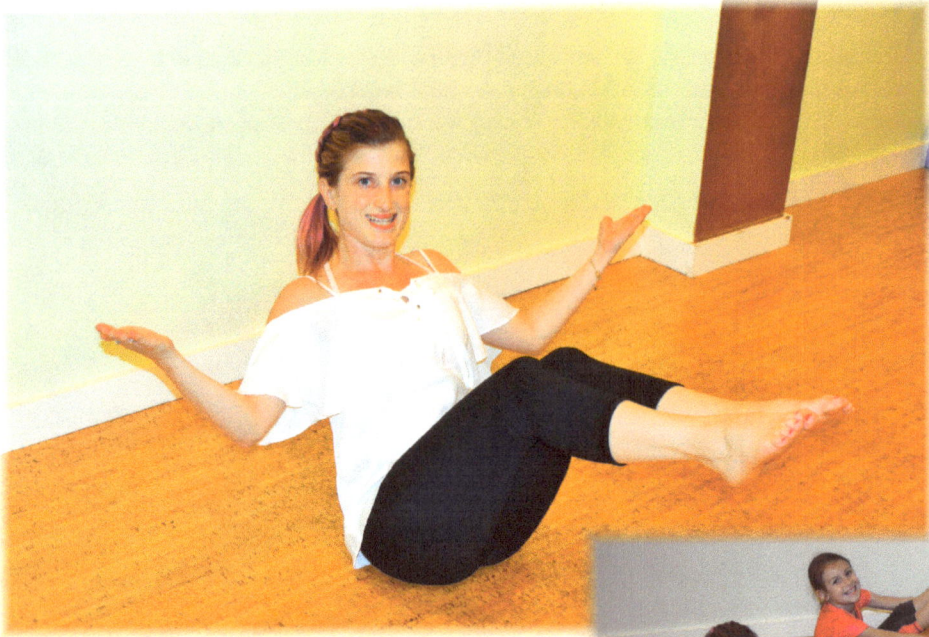

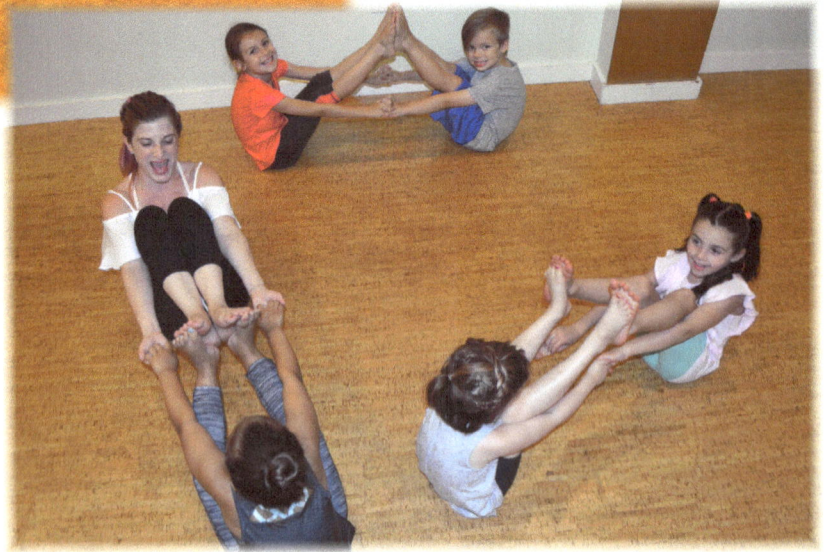

Let's sit up and pretend to be boats bobbing in the waves. Try lifting one leg at a time, finding your balance, and imagine rowing yourself downstream. Lift both legs and your arms to become a boat floating downstream.

Boat pose is a great core strengthener. It develops focus, stimulates the kidneys, and encourages digestion.

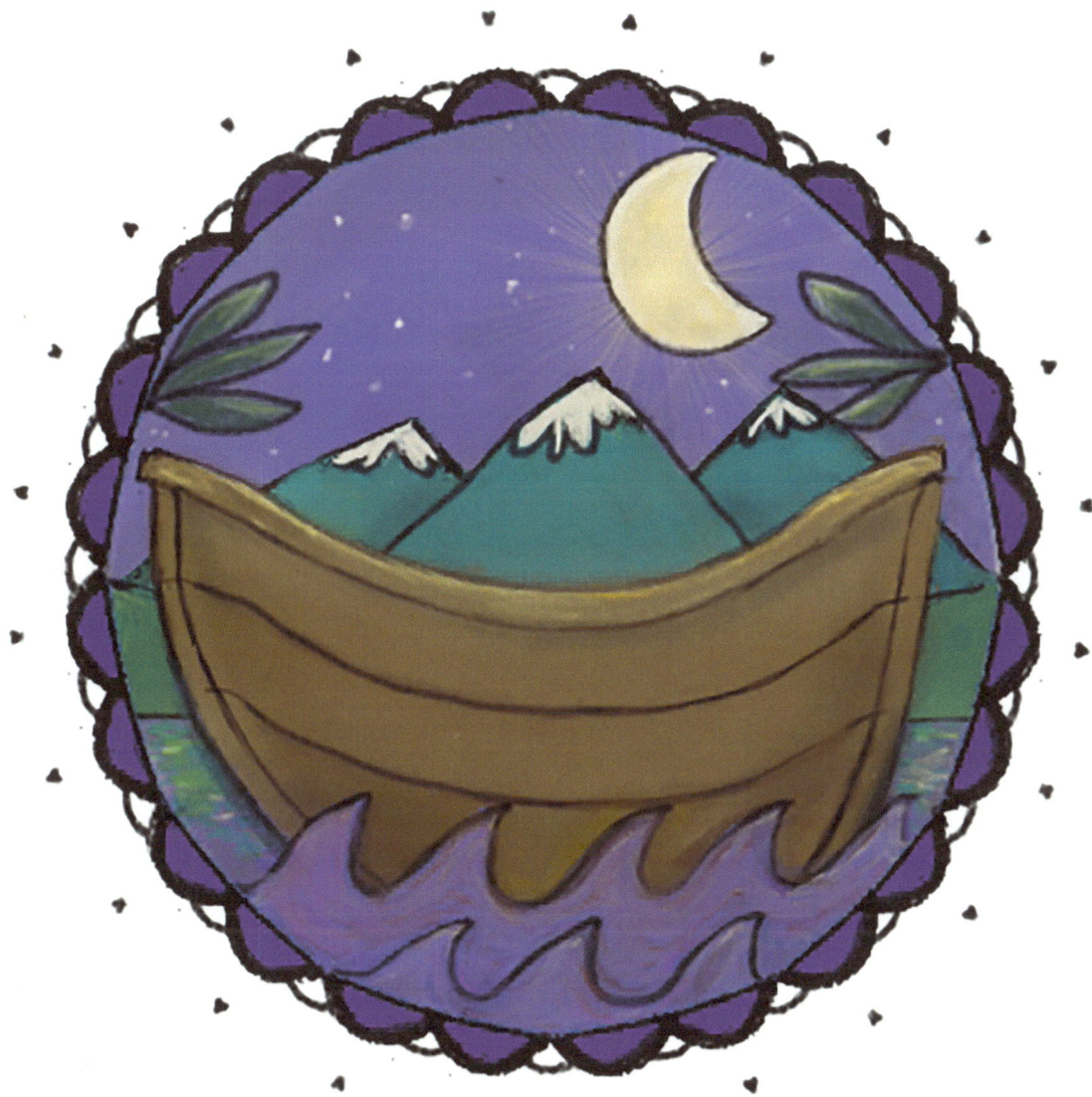

The next thing we did was hop into a boat,
and down that stream we went for a float,
and that little boat, oh that little boat,
that boat it looked like this.

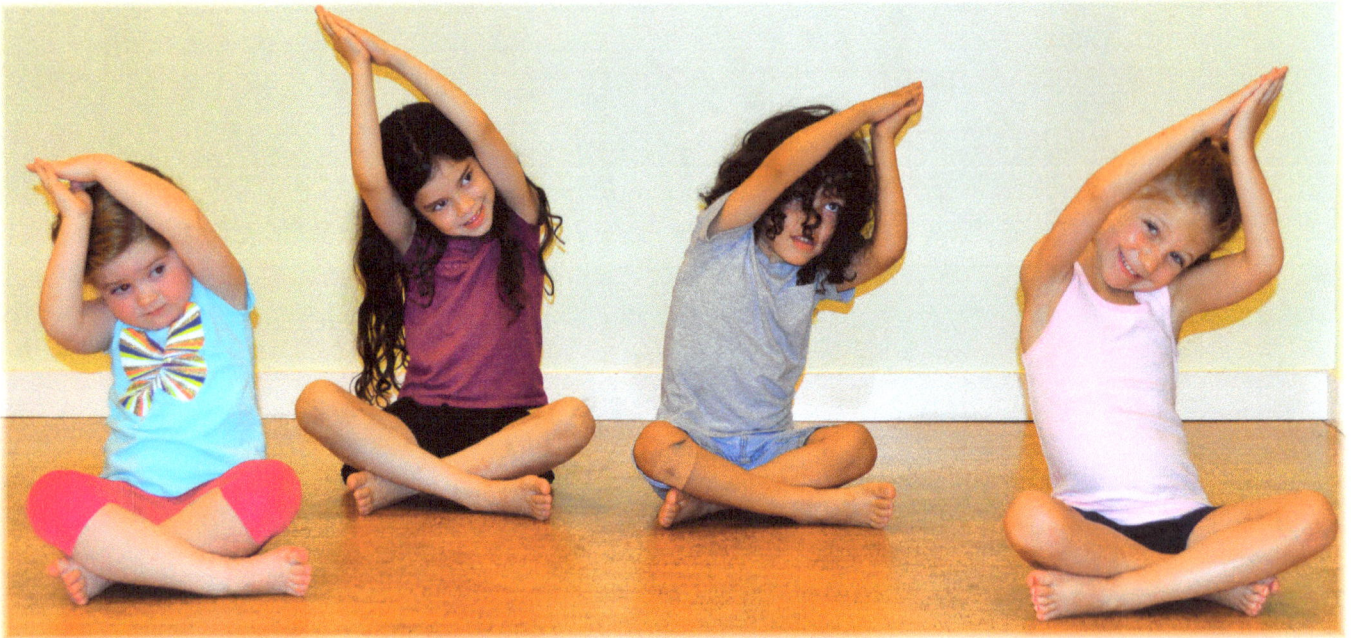

Seated on the floor, reach your arms up tall. Just a little higher and you might grab the moon! Bend to one side like a beautiful crescent moon. Tip to the other side and say hello to the stars.

This pose is a great stretch for the muscles on the sides of the body.

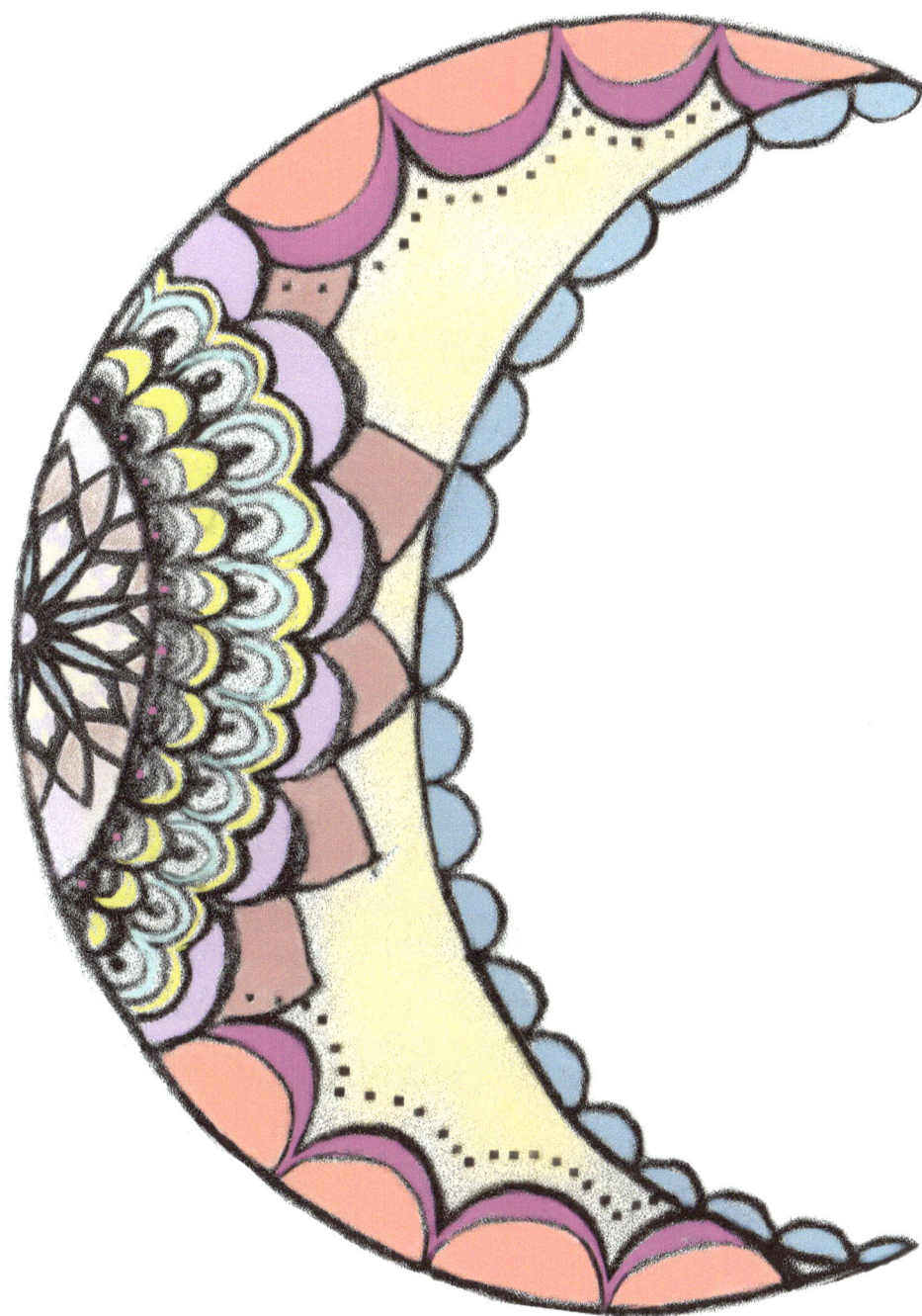

Our boat ride ended much too soon.
We were now floating by the light of the moon.
That moon up high, in the nighttime sky,
that moon it looked like this.

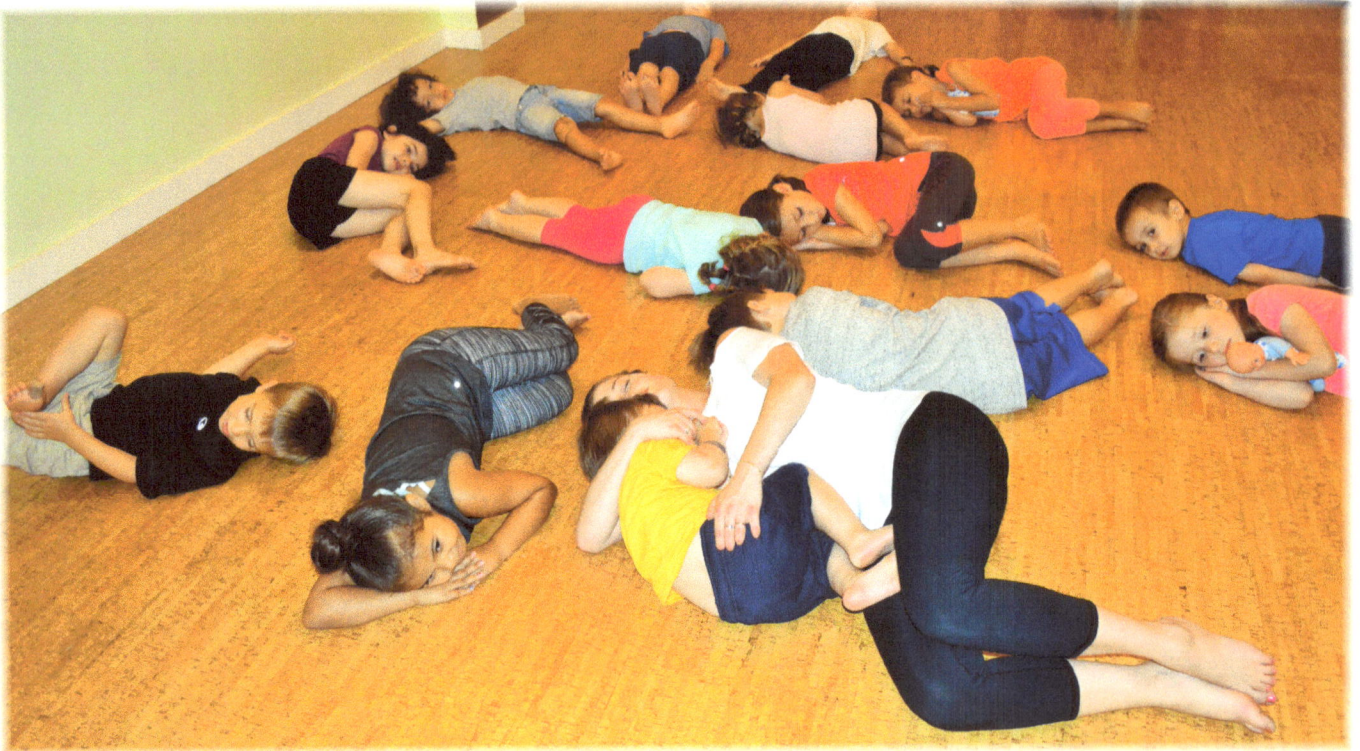

Lie on your back and close your eyes. Allow your arms to rest easily at your sides. Stretch your legs long and relax all of your muscles. Lie still and comfortable. Think about a blue sky and focus on the soft white clouds that float quietly by. Stay here for a few quiet minutes and rest.

This is known as Corpse pose. It relaxes the entire body and promotes a sense of calm. It can relieve stress and help encourage better sleep.

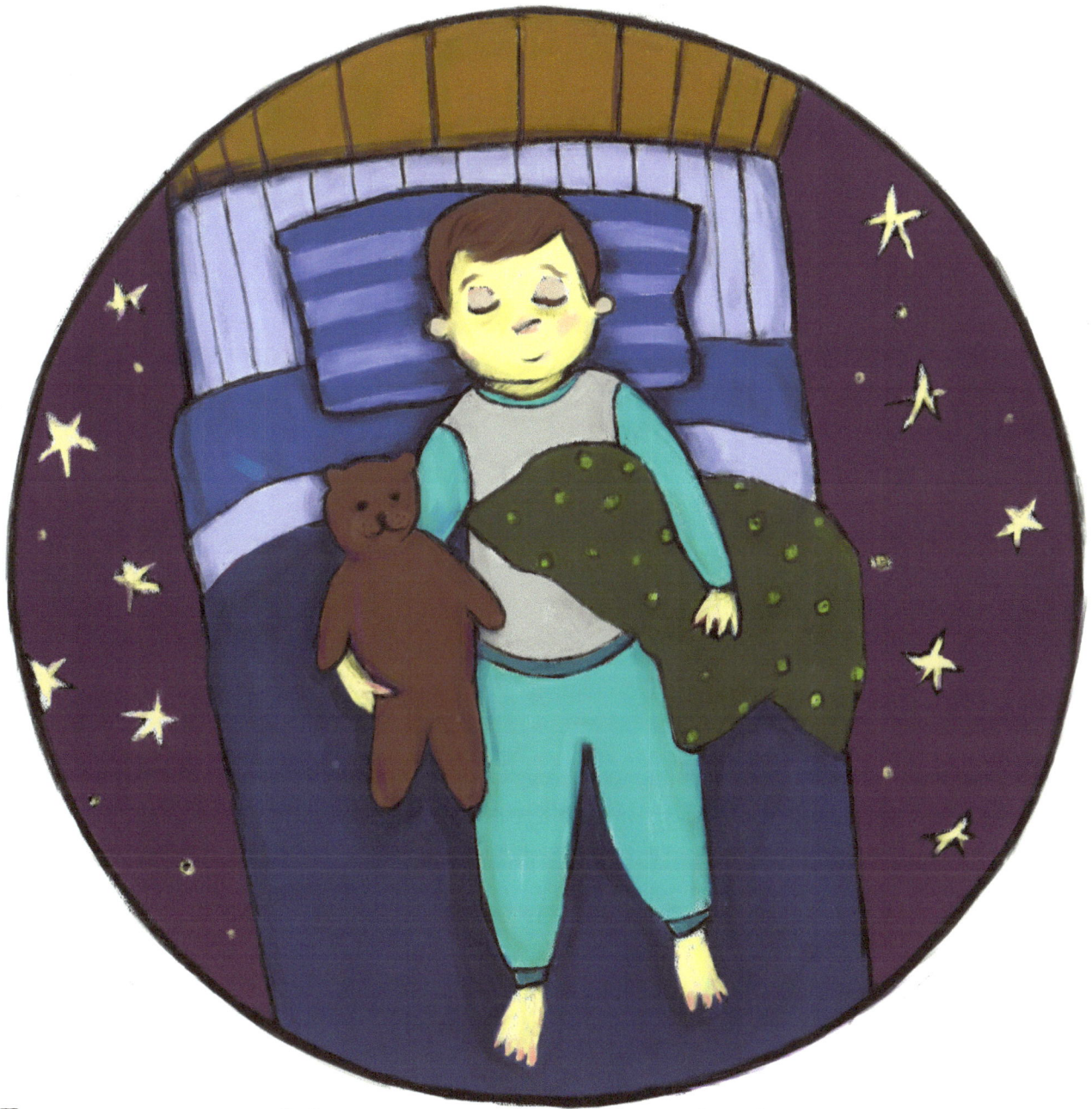

When we got home, we went straight to bed.
We were tired from the adventure we'd led.
We turned out the light and closed our eyes
tight, and slept all through the night.

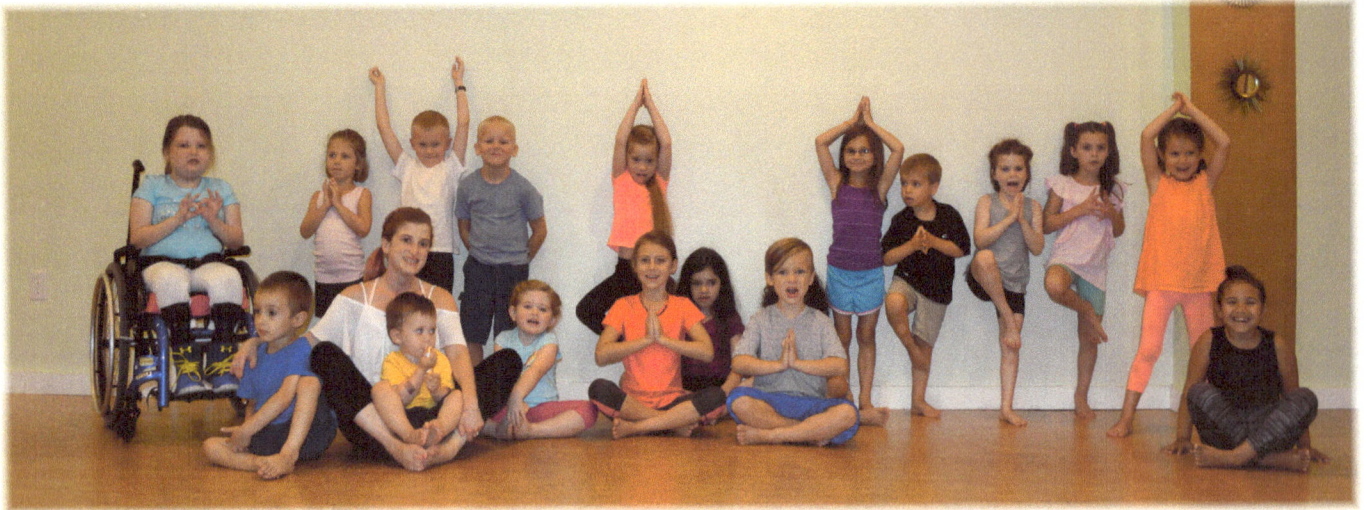

Thanks for joining us on our Yogaventure!

I hope you had as much fun as we did.

Visit www.JillianAmodio.com for a free Yogaventure song download and Yogaventure video!

You can use these next few pages to write or draw about other adventures you would like to take.

Maybe you can even come up with your very own yoga pose!

Namaste friends!